Beginner's Guide To Diet And Training

by

Paul Nam

For more works by this author, please visit:

Mobile Training Apps

www.pursefitness.com

Fitness Studio

www.theworkoutloft.com

Online Fitness Coaching

www.theworkoutloft.com/trainer-hack-see-results

PDF Books

https://payhip.com/wy2kool

OTHER BOOKS BY PAUL NAM

Available On Amazon

FIT TO FAT IN 8 WEEKS

SCRAWNY TO BRAWNY IN 8 WEEKS

NUTRITION 101: BUILDING THE FOUNDATION

IMMUNE SYSTEM 8: BOOST YOUR IMMUNE SYSTEM NATURALLY

IT'S ALL ABOUT YOUR HEALTH: FOOD RECIPES

THE BOOK OF CHOICES: THE LIVES OF 2 ATHLETES

BODYBUILDING AND STEROIDS: MY PERSONAL STORY

DUMBBELL TRAINING: FOR MEN AND WOMEN

DUMBBELL AND CORE TRAINING COMBINED: FOR MEN AND WOMEN

THE ULTIMATE GUIDE TO CORE(ABS) TRAINING: NO MORE LOW BACK PAIN

LEARN HOW TO STRETCH: FOR BETTER MOVEMENT AND HEALTH

TABLE OF CONTENTS

INTRODUCTION

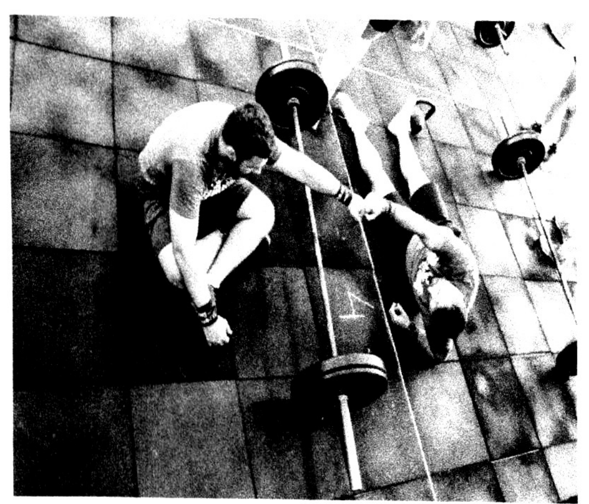

"Two more, yells your trainer." You grunt and push out two more repetitions on the bench press. You get up and look in the mirror. What you see back astonishes you. A lean and fit person who has been committed to the gym over the past year.

Committing yourself to the gym has not been an easy task. The past six months have been hell. Nothing went right. You did not lose weight, you injured your shoulder, and ran over your pet hamster with a lawn mower. To do this day you are baffled on how the hamster got outside.

This scenario happens to most people who start to an exercise regiment or the gym. I wish I knew the basics before I started to workout. My first bench press apparatus was a piano bench at the age of 17. I had no idea what I was doing but it felt awesome to lift weights. All I can remember is my chest swelling up after doing bench presses with my first barbell set. What an astonishing feeling that was.

Welcome to Beginner's Guide To Diet And Training. After reading this book, you will have the knowledge and confidence to start an exercise regiment.

UNDERSTANDING GENETIC LIMITATIONS

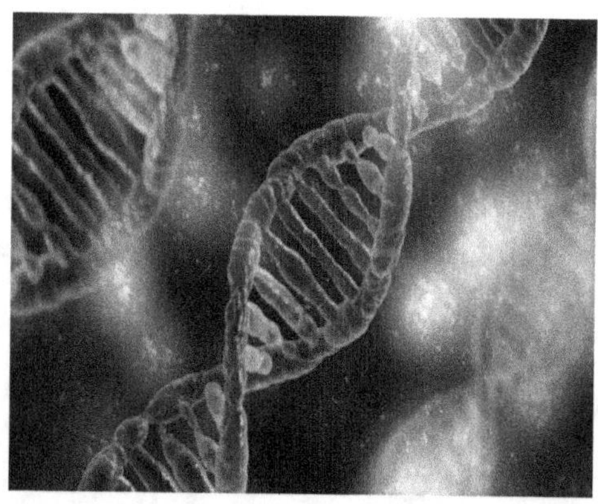

When you look at a fitness or bodybuilding magazine, what you see is a person who is chemically enhanced and has superior genetics. If a person looks like a super hero, there is a good chance they are using steroids, growth hormone, and other muscle building agents. I use to look like a super hero and it took a good amount of steroids to get there. I also trained very hard and had some decent genetics for bodybuilding.

What is genetics? Genetics are defined as the study of heredity, or how the characteristics of living things are transmitted from one generation to the next. Every living thing contains the genetic material that makes up DNA molecules. This material is passed on when organisms reproduce. The basic unit of heredity is the gene. What does that mean? That is the nerdy term. In a more simple term, it's what you are born with and what mother nature gave you to work with.

Understanding your own genetic limitations is the first step to building a physique that is attainable. Let's go over some basic body type structures. The three type of body structures I use to assess a person are ectomorph, mesomorph, and endomorph.

An ectomorph tends to be thin, and struggles to gain weight as either body fat or muscle. They can eat piles of food and stay looking the same, even when gaining muscular weight is their biggest goal. People who battle to gain muscle are often known as the typical hard gainer.

A mesomorph usually has a muscular chest and shoulders, muscular arms and legs, and minimal body fat. The put on muscle quickly but can gain body fat faster than an ectomorph. Most pro bodybuilders are mesomorphs.

The typical endomorph tends to gain weight and keep it on. Their build is a little wider than an ectomorph or mesomorph, with a thick ribcage, wide hips, and shorter limbs. They may have more muscle than either of the other body types, but they often struggle to gain it without significant amounts of accompanying body fat.

Now you have a basic understanding of the three different body types. Some people are often a mix of two different body types. For example, I am a mix of ectomorph and mesomorph. I can put on muscle fast but I am naturally skinny. Another person could be a mix of endomorph and mesomorph. A naturally muscular person who has wide hips and a slower metabolism.

Understanding what your body type is the first step to assessing how fast you can lose weight or achieve a physique that is attainable to you. Remember, the fitness models and bodybuilders you see in the magazines have superior genetics and use performance enhancing drugs. Pick a goal that is suitable for you to obtain naturally. If you are going to use performance enhancing drugs, educate yourself first. Any type of drug abuse can lead to serious health consequences.

HOW TO FIGURE OUT MACROS

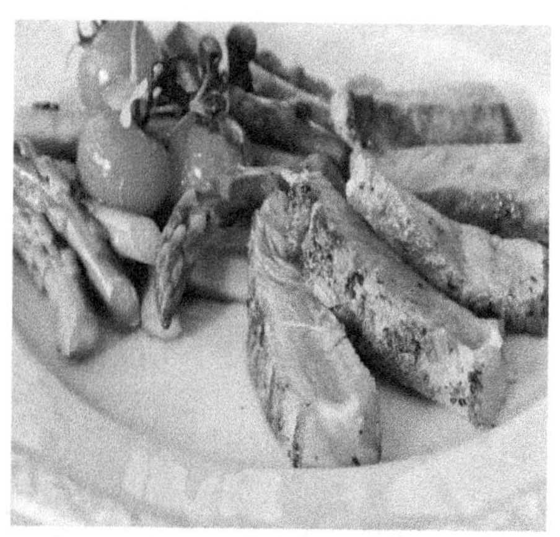

Nutrition. One of the most confusing aspects when it comes to fat loss, gaining muscle, and general fitness. Everyday we are bombarded with information on the media with the latest trends.

Here is a family friendly nutrition joke. What did the mother ghost tell the baby ghost when he ate too fast? Stop goblin your food. What a corny joke but it is nutrition related.

Before we start getting into the breakdown of the macro nutrients, let's go over the basics first. What is a macro nutrient? Macro nutrients are the largest class of nutrients the body requires and include protein, carbohydrates, and fats. Now let's get into the carbohydrates.

CARBOHYDRATES

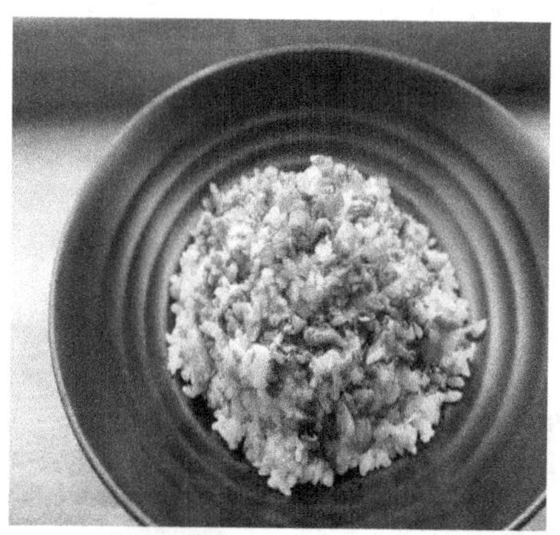

Oh, the love-hate relationship we have with carbs. Why do they taste so good? Carbohydrates are found in breads, fruit, rice, and even chocolate. There are many different types of carbohydrates, but the simplest types are called sugars. Throughout this chapter you'll learn about glucose, fiber, glycemic index, the role of insulin, and what is the recommended intake.

Glucose is made in the body to provide your body with energy, which is called adenosine triphosphate (ATP). This is the preferred energy source for your red blood cells. Glucose can also be converted to some amino acids, which are the building blocks of protein.

When your body needs energy, its first source is glucose. The body stores glucose inside your body as glycogen. The majority of glycogen is stored in your liver and skeletal muscle. When we need energy quickly, our bodies break down glycogen. This is important when understanding the basics of fat loss and muscle building.

As the general rule for fiber, humans can't digest it. Fiber contains certain bonds that our digestive system can't break down. The undigested fiber travels through our intestinal tract. Intestinal bacteria break down the fiber and other substances that are made by the bacteria. This process helps to nourish the cells that line our colon. This is why it's important to maintain healthy bacteria in our intestinal tract as this helps with the digestion process.

Fiber can found in vegetables, oats, legumes, rice, bran, seeds, soybean, and some fruits. It is important to include fiber in your daily diet. Many studies have shown that fiber can maintain health, prevent certain diseases, help to reduce blood cholesterol, and aid in weight management.

Understanding the glycemic response to foods is one way to help in the fight with fat loss. Glycemic response is the change in blood glucose after eating a certain type of food.

The Glycemic index (GI) is a rating system that's used to categorize foods. A food's glycemic index is a number that reflects the change in the blood glucose levels after it has been consumed. Foods with a GI higher than 70, such as potatoes, are considered high GI foods. Potatoes are high GI foods because after they're consumed, they cause a large increase in blood glucose levels. Foods such as beans, which have a glycemic index of 40 and lower, are considered a low GI food. This is because they cause a moderate rise in blood glucose levels. It is best to study and know the GI chart as this will give you the added advantage in losing fat or when it comes to building muscle.

The role of insulin in the body is very complex but understanding the basics will help with the way carbohydrates are absorbed and used for energy. Insulin is a hormone that's released by the pancreas in response to the rise in blood glucose levels that is caused by certain foods. This hormone helps with blood glucose regulation and energy storage. When a large, carbohydrate-based meal is eaten by itself, the pancreas releases insulin. Insulin in turn stimulates the excess glucose from the large carbohydrate meal into glycogen. The glycogen is then stored in the muscle and liver. When the muscle and liver are full, the excess glycogen is stored as fat. This is important to remember because if you constantly eat large amounts of carbohydrates and don't exercise enough, you may end up storing extra fat.

Most people wonder how many carbohydrates they really need in their diet. Carbohydrates are important energy source and some evidence has been shown that certain carbs may help to prevent chronic diseases. Good carbohydrate sources should come from whole grains, fruits, and vegetables. Man-made carbohydrates, like pasta, should be secondary and it's best to limit or eliminate refined sugars, such as candy.

There are certain recommendations and guidelines to follow when it comes to carbohydrate consumption. A general guideline and acceptable macro nutrient range is 45% - 65% of your total caloric intake. So, if a person consumes 2,500 calories in a day, they would eat 281-406 grams of carbohydrates per day. This macro nutrient has 4 calories per gram. In order to get the proper range, you would times .45 by 2,500, then divide by 4, and this would equal 281. Next, you would do .65 times 2,500, and then divide by 4, which would equal 406. If you were to eat 6 small meals a day, your carb intake would be 47-68 grams per meal. To get those numbers all you would have to do is divide 281 and

406 by 6. Added sugars should be no more than 25% of your total calories. Also, it's recommended that adults consume at least 14 grams of fiber daily.

My only carbohydrate sources are fruit, vegetables, and steel cut oats. I rarely eat carbohydrates such as rice, bread, and pasta. This is from years of following a low carbohydrate diet. I feel good every day and I try to maintain a 9-10% bodyfat year round.

If you are unsure of other carbohydrate recommendations, feel free to visit the My Pyramid website at http://www.pyramid.gov.

PROTEINS

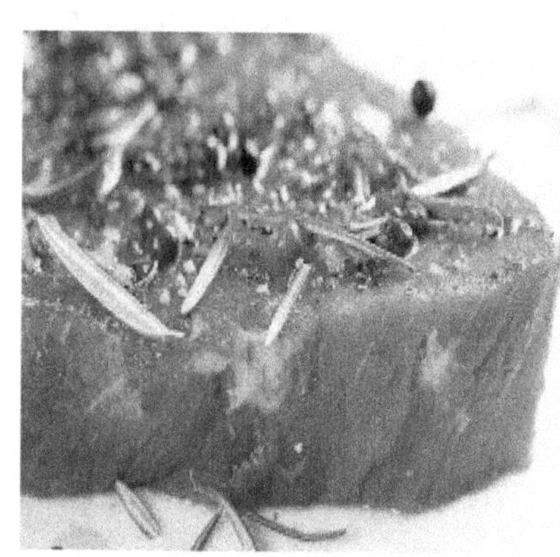

Steak. Chicken. Tuna. Many people relate protein to a muscle building nutrient, but the term protein was derived more than 170 years ago from the Greek word "prota", meaning of primary importance.

Proteins are macro molecules and are made up of smaller units called amino acids. They are formed together by special chemical bonds called peptide bonds. Some proteins are simple and contain only a few amino acids while others can have 250 to 300 different amino acids.

Our bodies need 20 different amino acids to be complete and in good health. These amino acids are called essential, nonessential, or conditionally essential. The 11 amino acids that can be made from other sources are called the nonessential amino acids. The other 9 amino acids and called essential because your body cannot make them from other sources and must be obtained from food.

Some foods have more protein than others or have a different combination of amino acids. An example would be a slice of white bread versus a whole egg. Both contain protein, but the egg has more nutritional value than the bread. The reason is because the egg is a complete protein and the bread is an incomplete protein. A complete protein is a source of protein that contains an adequate proportion of all nine of the essential amino acids necessary for the dietary needs of humans. Incomplete proteins are foods that contain very small amounts of one or more of the essential amino acids. Meat, eggs, and dairy products are complete sources of protein. Plant and plant products are considered incomplete protein sources and by combining 2 incomplete protein sources you can a make a complete protein.

Protein quality is determined by how your body absorbs and digests the amino acids in the protein. High quality proteins are complete protein sources with good amino acid bio availability. Low quality sources are incomplete protein sources or one that has poor amino acid bio availability. Bio availability is defined as the proportion of a nutrient that is absorbed from the diet and used for normal body functions.

When we eat protein, it's broken down and circulates throughout the body, contributing to many types of bodily functions such as movement, regulating pH balance, protection, and energy. Protein also provides structure towards your muscles, skin, bone, hair, and fingernails. Proteins are also an important component of your cell membrane and structure. Consider them the building blocks of the entire body.

We walk, swim, run, and get out of bed every morning. Protein is needed for movement when it comes to the relaxation and contraction of the muscles in the human body. There are 3 types of muscles in your body: skeletal muscle, cardiac muscle, and smooth muscle. About half of the body's protein is present in your skeletal muscle so eating enough protein is important factor in maintaining your muscle mass. Not getting the required amount of protein in your diet will slow down your recovery time after an intense weight training session.

Internally, proteins are needed for protection from physical dangers and infections. Your skin is made up of protein and it serves as a barrier to the outside and inside environment. When people cut themselves, a blood clot forms to stop the outside bacteria from entering. The specific protein that causes this blood clot is called fibrinogen. Your immune system also produces proteins if an infection enters the body. The immune system will also produce antibodies to help fight off the infection.

People who are protein deficient lack the necessary tools to fight of infections so they get sick more often.

Proteins can be used as an energy source also when your energy levels are low. Your body first turns stored glycogen then to fatty acids as an energy source. When these 2 storage areas are low, your body then utilizes some amino acids into energy.

Remember that carbohydrates and proteins give your body 4 kcal of energy while fats give you 9 kcals of energy per 1 gram. This important to remember when you're trying to lose body fat, as not eating enough carbs and fats can contribute to muscle mass loss.

How much protein do we really need? Protein requirements are usually divided into 2 segments, sedentary and active. For the typical sedentary male, it's recommended he consume 80-90 grams per day. For a sedentary female it is recommended she eat 60-70 grams a day. So the sedentary male should eat 3 meals a day at 26.6-30 grams per meal and the female should have 20-23.3 grams per meal. For people who follow a regular exercise regiment they would have 1.6 to 2.2 grams kg/day. A person weighing 160 lbs. would be 72.7 in kilograms (160/2.2). The person would consume between 116grams (72.7x1.6) and 160grams (72.7x2.2) per day. A person who is physically active generally eats 3 meals and 2 snacks so that would work out to 23.2grams (116/5) and 32 grams (160/5) per meal. Females would consume the smaller amount, which is 116 grams, and males would consume the higher amount, which is 160 grams.

As a percentage guideline, you can eat 10-35% of your energy as protein. So a person who eats 2,500 calories a day would consume between 62.5 grams (2,500x.10/4) and 219 grams (2,500x.35/4). If you were to eat 5 small meals a day, you would eat 12.5 grams(62.5/5) or 43.8 grams(219/5) per each meal. The females would stay at the lower range and males at the upper range.

FATS

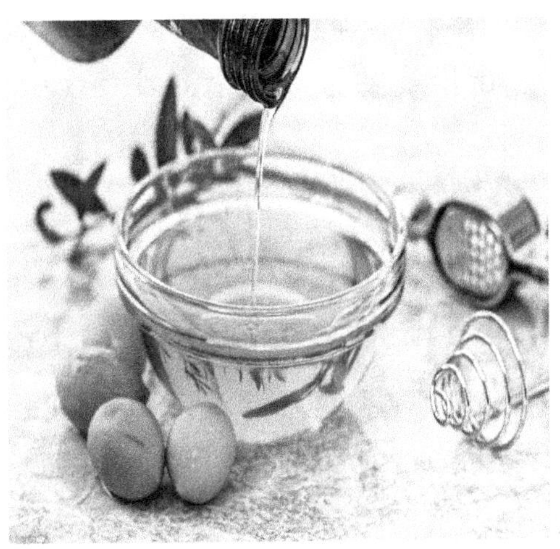

As we know, most fats are unhealthy, but some are actually good for you. Did you ever wonder why peanut butter taste so good? Fats can be naturally found in foods but if they are consumed in high amounts they can contribute to obesity.

People watching their caloric intake often buy fat-free foods in order to lose weight or follow a specific diet. Some companies have even come out with fat substitutes in order to replace the fats we normally eat in foods.

Fats are 9 calories per gram and they provide a major source of energy for the body. Fats and oils are also known as Lipids. Lipids that are liquid at room temperature are called oils. Lipids that are solid at room temperature are called fats. Saturated fatty acids are solid at room temperature and can be found in butter, beef, and animal products. The shorter form of saturated fatty acids is called saturated fat and that is a more common name to the general public. Trans fatty acids tend to be solid at room temperature and are found in foods such as dairy and beef products. Most trans fatty acids are produced by a process called partial hydrogenation. This process converts oily lipids into solid fats by changing their structure. Processed food contains large amounts of trans fatty acids. Companies use trans fatty acids so that their foods look more desirable for consumption and it helps to reduce food spoilage. Always try to limit the amount of processed foods you eat because of the high amounts of trans fatty acids. There could be a link between eating this type of fat and developing cardiovascular disease.

There are so many different types of fats that most people wonder which ones are really important. The 2 essential fatty acids our bodies really need are linoleic acid and linolenic acid.

Linoleic acid is known as omega 6 fatty acid and linolenic acid is known as omega 3 fatty acid.

Omega 3 and 6 are essential nutrients because they are needed by the body but cannot be processed in sufficient amounts to meet our body's needs. They have several functions in the body, but omega 3 fatty acids help to reduce inflammation, and helps to relax the blood vessel walls. This may help to reduce the risk of cardiovascular disease. Most people get enough omega 6 in their diets but usually not enough omega 3 fatty acids.

Most foods we eat contain some form of fatty acids. Nuts, seeds, and certain oils such as soybean, or corn have a good amount of omega 6 fats. Other oils that are made from canola, soybean, and flax seed have omega 3 fats. Some foods such as soybean oil, and walnuts contain both sources of both essential fatty acids. In today`s society we generally have access to all these foods so getting enough of these 2 types of fats should not be an issue. Just remember to follow one simple rule, eat more omega 3 than 6.

Now let`s move on to the saturated and unsaturated fatty acids. Our bodies can make most saturated and unsaturated fatty acids so they are not essential in the diet. We get most of our saturated fats from eating animal fats and we get most get most our unsaturated fats from eating vegetables and plants.

Fats can also be used for an energy source in a form called triglycerides. When being compared to protein and carbohydrates, fats yield the highest amount of energy. When fat is broken down, it gives the body 9 kcal of energy per 1 gram. Proteins and carbohydrates give the body 4 kcal of energy per 1 gram. This is important to remember, as we get into the fat loss and energy equations in the upcoming chapters. Your body has to have low insulin levels and has to be in a semi-starvation state in order for fat to be used as an energy source. Exercise and physiological stress can help to burn fat when your body is in the semi-starvation state.

Fatty acids can also be turned into ketones by a process called ketogenesis, which can only happen when blood glucose levels are low. The brain, heart, skeletal muscle, and the kidneys can use ketones. During times of severe low glycogen levels, the body can use ketones first for energy instead of using protein, which is located inside of the muscle cells. Your body is not in a good state when it starts to break down muscle tissue for energy. This is detrimental for both fat loss and muscle building.

When a person does not need any more energy, it stores the excess fatty acids into their fat cells and then into their skeletal muscle. Adipose tissue contains special cells called adipocytes, which can store large amounts of fats. Fat tissues are found around your vital organs, which are called visceral adipose tissue. Fat tissues that are found underneath your skin are called subcutaneous adipose tissue.

Insulin is a powerful hormone in our body and is responsible for the storage of fatty acids during times of excess energy intake. Insulin causes your fatty tissues to take up glucose and fatty acids. It also helps to convert excess glucose to fatty acids. Understanding the role of insulin in our body will help you to lose those extra pounds or help to gain those few pounds of muscle.

As some people know already low-density lipoproteins are known as the bad cholesterol. LDL can build up of a substance called plaque on the vessel walls. This plaque can build up slowly over time and even block blood flow, which may lead to a condition called cardiovascular disease. Eating high amounts of saturated fatty acids, trans fats, and cholesterol can increase the buildup of LDL in your blood. To lower your LDL concentration, eat a diet with more polyunsaturated fatty acids (fatty fish), omega 3 fats, and fiber.

The liver produces high-density lipoprotein, which circulate in the blood to collect the excess cholesterol from your cells. HDL is known as the good cholesterol. There may be some evidence showing that having higher levels of HDL may reduce the risk of cardiovascular disease. Eating a low carbohydrate diet, monounsaturated fatty acids (such as olive oil), and consuming moderate amounts of alcohol, may contribute to higher levels of HDL in the human body. So just remember to eat more foods with HDL and less foods with LDL.

Fats are 9 calories per gram and eating them in excess can contribute to obesity. Obesity is not only a major health concern but now is a global problem. Obesity may increase the chances of cardiovascular disease, type 2 diabetes, and even some forms of cancer. A simple rule to remember is to limit the consumption of foods that are high in fat as they contain the most calories.

Food companies have developed fat substitutes in order for people to eat low fat foods. These are made from carbohydrates, proteins, and a blend of carbohydrates and fatty acids. Olestra is an example of a fat substitute made from sucrose and some fatty acids. Other examples are Maltrin and Stellar, which are made from carbohydrates and proteins. Fat free does not mean calorie free as both carbs and protein are 4 calories per gram.

So remember that next time you buy fat-free foods as they will be reduced in calories but not completely free of them.

Eating enough essential fatty acids in your diet is important for your overall health. It is recommended for omega 6 fats you eat only 12 grams to 17 grams a day for both male and female adults. For omega 3 fats it is recommended that you have 2 servings of foods that are high in omega 3 fats daily. You should always limit your intake of saturated fats as eating them in excess may lead to cardiovascular disease. The recommended intake for saturated fats is 10% of total calories consumed in day. So at 2000 calories, 10 percent would be 200 (2000x.10) calories and 22.2 (200/9) grams per day. Trans fatty acids that are commercially produced should be limited to 1% of your total food intake for the day. Cholesterol should be limited to 300mg daily and this is equal to 2 whole eggs. The total amount of fats an adult should consume is 20% to 35% of your total calories consumed for the day. A person eating 2,500 calories in a day that would be 500 calories (2,500x0.2) and 875 calories (2,500x0.35) which is 55.6 grams (500/9) and 97.2

grams (875/9). If you were to eat 5 small meals a day, you would eat 11.12 grams(55.6/5) or 19.4 grams (97.2/5) per meal.

I take omega 3 capsules year round for a healthy heart and for good cardiovascular health. I also eat cheese, nuts, and use extra olive oil virgin oil for salad dressings.

The best sources of fats come from fatty fish, omega 3, flax seed oil, nuts, seeds, extra virgin olive oil, avocados, and cheese.

GUIDELINES FOR WEIGHT TRAINING

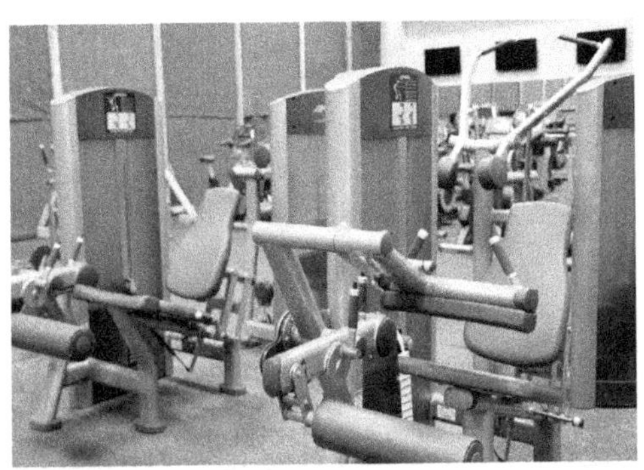 Walking into a weight room or gym can be intimidating if you have no direction or knowledge on how to use the equipment. You often see 2 types of people in the gym. The buff people and the people who are trying to get fit. The buff people have perfect form and look like pros when they train. The people who are trying to get fit look like they are doing exercises from a different planet. Which one would you like to be? The obvious answer is the fit person who knows what they are doing but we do not live in a perfect world.

Here are some guidelines to get you started.

1. Always practice good form. A good controlled set will recruit more muscle fibers verses throwing the weights around.

2. Do one warm up set with a lighter weight. This will allow you to practice the exercise and execute good form for the next sets.

3. Lower the weight in a controlled manner. The lowering part of the rep is called the negative (eccentric) portion. More control in the lowering portion will recruit more muscle fibers.

4. Breathe out with force. Never hold your breath during a set. Your muscles need oxygen to keep working and to expel carbon dioxide. A red face does not look attractive.

5. Know when to stop. Sometimes it is not good to push beyond failure. Pushing yourself too hard all the time can lead to injuries.

6. Record your weights in a book to track your progress. This is how to track your progress.

7. Do large muscle groups before smaller muscle groups as they require the most energy. Doing biceps before training your back is detrimental to your back workout as your arms will fatigue first.

8. Always set goals before you start any training program. Whether it be to lose 5lb, 10lbs, or to bench press your body weight. This will give you more purpose and will help you reach your goal.

9. Try not to grunt or scream when you do your set or reps. You're not auditioning for Tarzan.

10. If you are unsure of any exercises just look them up in the internet. Just use Google.

11. Have a protein shake or meal within 1 hour after training. This will help to replenish your glycogen levels and rebuild the torn muscle. Eat a carbohydrate and protein source.

12. Never eat right before your workout. This will cause an upset stomach and result in a horrible workout. It is best to wait 1-1.5 hours.

13. It is best to weight train at least 2-3x a week. You want to hit each body part at least once a week. If you are doing full body workouts, 2-3x a week is optimal. More is not better. Your body needs to rest.

GUIDELINES FOR CARDIO

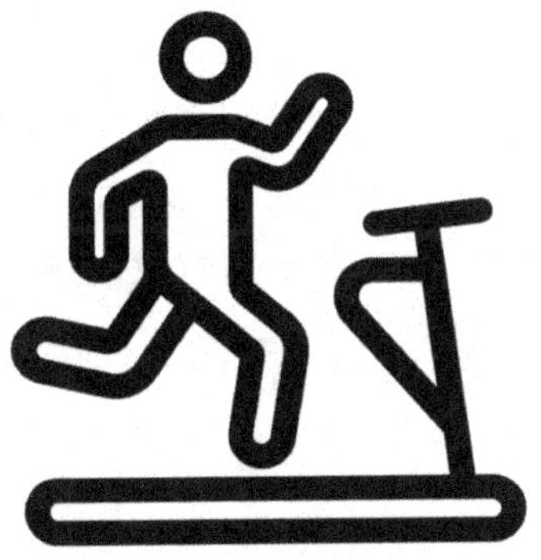 Cardiovascular workouts are great for your lungs and heart. These types of workouts help you to get into shape by burning those extra calories.

I teach a success equation to all my clients. This equation has 3 components to it. The 3 components are nutrition, cardio, and weight training. Each component equals 100 percent results. The cardio component is around 20-30 percent of the equation. Cardio is an important part of exercise. I use to hate it but now I look forward to my cardio sessions.

Here are some tips to get you started.

1. Never do cardio on a full stomach. It is best to do cardio after 1-.1.5 hours after eating.

2. Do cardio at least 2-3x a week. If you are just going to cardio workouts without any weight training, aim for 4-5 times a week.

3. Always warm up before increasing your intensity. A 5 minute warm up is usually suitable. When doing higher intensity, make sure you can carry on a conversation while exercising. This is called the "talk test".

4. Exercise for at least 20 minutes at a time. Then move up to 30 minutes. When 30 minutes is no longer a challenge, go up to 40 minutes.

5. Do cardio exercises which you enjoy and are suitable for your body type. This will make exercising not seem like a chore. If you do an exercise that is not suitable for your body type, an injury could occur.

GUIDELINES FOR STRETCHING

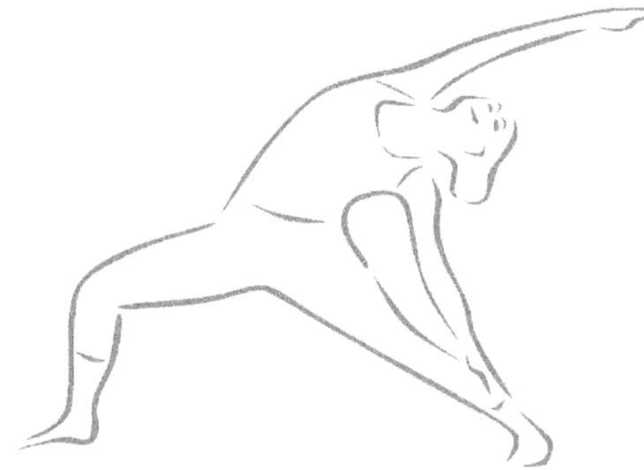 Our bodies are designed for movement. We walk, run to catch that late bus, swim, and use movement to shovel the snow off our driveways. There are many reasons why we should stretch, but the number reason is to increase your flexibility.

Flexibility is defined as movement in a joint or series of joints, and length in muscles that cross the joints to induce a bending movement or motion. If your not flexible, everyday movements become harder to do.

I stretch 5 days a week and with my clients everyday. I should get a medal for this achievement but let's get into the guidelines.

Here are some guidelines to get you started.

1. Always do static stretching after you exercise. This helps with recovery an improves the range of motion.

2. Hold a static stretch for 10-30 seconds.

3. Always do a dynamic stretch before you exercise. This warms up the area so there is less chance of injury.

4. Always do a dynamic stretch before you exercise. When doing a dynamic stretch, move the area for 10-30 seconds.

5. Never hold your breath when you stretch. People will think you have high blood pressure and they might call 911. In Yoga, you breathe with the stretch.

6. Never stretch a cold muscle. This could lead to an injury. Always warm up first.

7. Never stretch or exercise on a full stomach. Unless you enjoy expelling unpleasant air which will kill people at the gym.

8. Never push the stretch past the point of the normal range of motion. Only do this with a qualified professional or if you have done it before.

9. If you feel pain when you stretch, just stop. Always listen to your body.

SETTING GUIDELINES: CUTTING OR BULKING

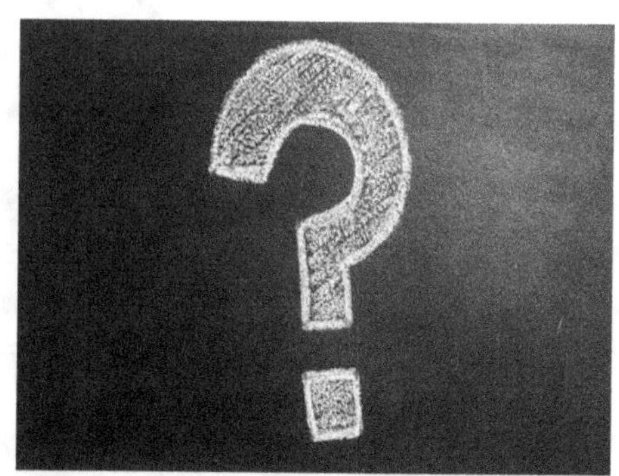

Going back to setting goals, it is always important to establish what you want to accomplish before committing to the gym. Do you want to lose body fat, gain muscle, or get fit? In reality, we wish we could do all 3. In order to do this you would have to do anabolic steroids and a host of other performance enhancing drugs. In the end, it is not worth it.

For example, when I use to prepare for a bodybuilding show, I would have a bulking and cutting phase. During my bulking phase my caloric intake was very high and I would focus was on lifting heavy weights. The type of steroids I used were meant for pure muscle mass. I won't go into detail about my steroid usage. You can read that information in my other book called Bodybuilding And Steroids: My Personal Story. The end result would be a bulky Asian with an extra 20 lbs of muscle and fat.

After feeling bloated and looking a state puff marshmallow, I would plan the cutting phase for my competition. My diet would be very restrictive and my focus was on implementing more cardio into my routine. The one thing I hated. I also switched the type of steroids I was using. The type of steroids I used were meant for cutting and preserving my muscle mass. The main point is through bodybuilding drugs, I could retain 80-85% of my muscle mass, while I dieted. If I did this process naturally with just supplements, I would retain only 60% or less of my muscle mass.

By being a trainer for over 20 years and helping people reach their goals, it is best to pick one goal and pursue it. Sure you can have a smaller goal within that goal, but stick to one for the best results. If you want to bulk, just bulk. If you want to cut, eat and train towards getting cut.

LEARNING THE PROPER WAY TO GET CUT

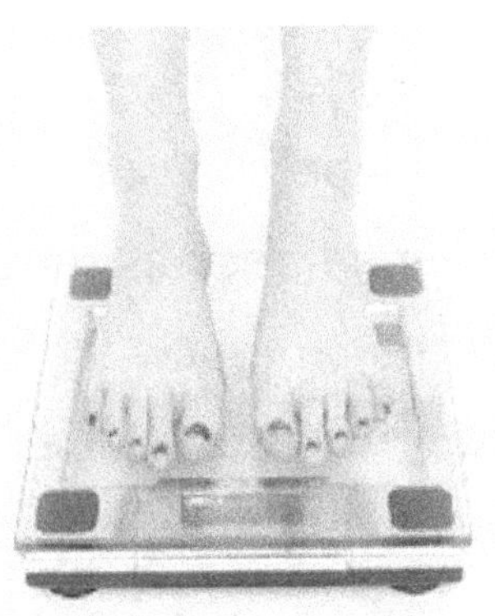

Drink this miracle shake and lose 10 lbs? We all hear these miracle claims over social media. I wish it was that easy to lose body fat. In reality, it does take work to get cut. It takes work to become rich, to build that dream house, and to have a stable relationship. There is a wrong way and right way. Let's get started on the right way.

Why do we need to eat?

Humans need to eat in order to have energy for every day movements. What happens when a person's every movement becomes limited because of a sedentary job or an injury? The go into a positive energy balance develop adipose tissue(fat cells).

Adipose tissue is made up of lipid-filled cells called adipocytes, which contain a core of triglycerides. The number and size of adipocytes determine the mass of adipose in a person's body. If a person is in consistent positive energy balance, their adipocytes start to fill up with triglyceride. When that adipocyte if full, a new one is formed and the process continues. When a person loses body fat, the enlarged adipocyte shrinks back to normal size but the number of adipocytes remain the same. This is why when a person loses 20 lbs from following a successful weight loss plan, they gain the weight back fast as soon as they go back to eating junk food and larger food portions.

Inside the human body, adipose tissue is found throughout the body. Visceral adipose tissue (VAT) is defined as tissue deposited between the internal organs and the abdominal area. Subcutaneous adipose tissue (SCAT) is adipose tissue that is found beneath the skin. VAT is considered more of a health risk than SCAT because the intra-abdominal fat is more likely to undergo lipolysis. Lipolysis is the breakdown of a triglyceride molecule into glycerol and fatty acids.

This may cause an increase in levels of LDL (bad) cholesterol, insulin, and a decrease in HDL (good) cholesterol. Other conditions such as high blood pressure, type 2 diabetes, and inflammation may become more prevalent due to having excessive intra-abdominal fat.

Overeating and inactivity are 2 main causes that contribute to obesity. We now know that being in a consistent positive energy balance can make a person gain adipose tissue. There are many societal and physiological factors that can influence the amount of food a person eats.

Two can dine for $6.99? Who could say no to such a deal? But what we don't all know is that this popular value meal can pack 1350 calories (for one person), which is more than half of the daily energy requirements. These types of fast foods are energy dense, inexpensive, readily available, and accepted as the cultural norm. Societal influence can affect the amount and what type of food people eat. We often see advertisements and commercials every day for these types of food. Studies have also shown that people tend to eat more if the serving size is larger. Do you think about portion size when you go to an all you can eat buffet? I try not go to all you can eat buffets as it usually ends in stomach ache from over eating.

Obesity can also result from having poor self-esteem. Eating food can make a person feel good and some people eat to cope with stress. Obese individuals may experience depression and panic attacks more than people who are at a normal weight. A person's social network may also affect if they gain weight or not. If all of your friends eat fast food all the time and do not exercise, there is a good chance you will do the same.

Eating for fat loss can be one of the most challenging and confusing aspects, since there are so many so-called experts out there with different opinions on fat loss. After training over 1000 people and competing in over 20 bodybuilding shows, I have formulated my own recipe for success that requires some simple steps.

The first step is to figure out a person's BMR. To figure out your BMR, google BMR calculator and put in your height, age, and weight. A male who is 35 years old, 172 cms, weighs 165 lbs and has an BMR of 1706 kcal per day. So he would need at least 1706 kcal per day to maintain normal body functions at rest. Next step is to figure out his caloric intake using a calorie counting app like MyFitnessPal or an online counting system. If he has a BMR of 1706 kcal per day and is ingesting over 2400 calories per day, he would be in a positive energy balance. In order to lose body fat, he would then have to exercise to burn off those extra calories.

Exercising can consist of cardiovascular or resistance workouts, or a combination of both. A combination of both is recommended as they both burn calories and work different areas.

Cardiovascular workouts are good for your heart, lungs, and VO2 max while resistance training is good for building muscle mass. As we have learned earlier, muscle mass burns more calories at rest. So, if he did 2 cardiovascular workouts and burned 300 calories at each session, then he completed 2 resistance-training workouts and burned 200 calories at each, the total calories burned would be 1000 calories for the week, putting him at 1400 (2400-1000) calories for the week. Remember, he has a BMR of 1706 kcal per day and this would put him in a negative energy balance (1400-1706) where weight loss would occur. If he was to ingest 2800 calories a day and did not want to give up some junk food, I would suggest for him to lengthen the duration of the workouts to burn off those extra calories. Our bodies do not like extreme changes as it works to maintain homeostasis all the time.

If you follow your BMR and exercise, you will lose weight. I have used TDEE and other equations but found this was the fastest route to fat loss. If you have a hard time following your BMR, follow these 3 steps first to lighten up your caloric intake. There are 3 things you need to cut gradually back on which are sugars, carbohydrates, and certain fats. Sugars and carbohydrates both raise your insulin levels and this promotes fat storage. Fats are 9 calories per gram so cutting back will automatically lighten up a person's caloric intake. Just remember a simple rule, eat more omega 3 fats. Another rule I use is not to eat sugars or carbohydrates after 6 pm. When a person wakes up they burn carbohydrates as a fuel source because their glycogen levels are low but at night carbohydrates are stored for later use. If you are hungry at night eat a small portion of protein and vegetables or just protein by itself. Just make sure you don't eat a 12-ounce steak before you go to bed, as anything in excess will be turned into body fat.

If you are eating well over your BMR and cannot cut your calories that drastic, use the TDEE first. Figure out what your TDEE is and then follow that number. Once you stop losing body-fat, use the BMR next.

Should I eat every 2 or 3 hours and how many meals should I eat in a day? Meal timing and portion size is a crucial component when it comes to burning fat. Some experts say 3 meals and day and 2 snacks. Others say 3 meals and 3 protein s hakes a day. There is no perfect system to lose weight but what I usually recommend 3 meals and 1-2 snacks a day. If my clients are eating close to their BMR and feel full I do not add extra calories to their meals as they may cause unwanted weight gain. I work with what they already eat and I just recommend healthier food choices. People who have kids and a full time job do not have time to eat 5-6 times a day. As for meal timing usually 2.5-3 hours between all meals or snacks will give the intestinal tract enough time to digest the food. The goal here is to figure out what works for you, as your metabolism is different from other people. What should I eat for a snack? I usually eat a 5 oz. protein serving with 1 cup of natural yogurt before I go to bed. This snack does not raise my insulin levels and keeps me full. Other good snack choices are natural cheese, Greek yogurt, small handful of nuts, vegetables and hummus, low carbohydrate protein bars, and slower-releasing protein powder. Another quick snack would be the meat leftovers from your supper.

TRAINING TIPS WHEN CUTTING

Here are some training tips to get you started on your journey when training to get cut.

1. Increase your calorie deficit with cardio. Just do more cardiovascular workouts. Mix up your cardio for best results.

2. Train in the am if you can. You will burn more body fat since your glycogen levels are lower in the morning.

3. Do more full body workouts. These types of workouts burn more calories which lead to faster fat loss.

4. Take less rest in between sets and reps. This will increase your heart rate which will burn more calories. Instead of 40-60 seconds rest periods, cut it down to 20-30 seconds.

5. Use supersets to increase the intensity of the workout which will result in extra calories burned. A

superset is when one set of an exercise is performed directly after a set of a different exercise without rest between them. Once each superset is complete, then rest for 40-60 seconds to recover.

LEARNING THE PROPER WAY TO BULK

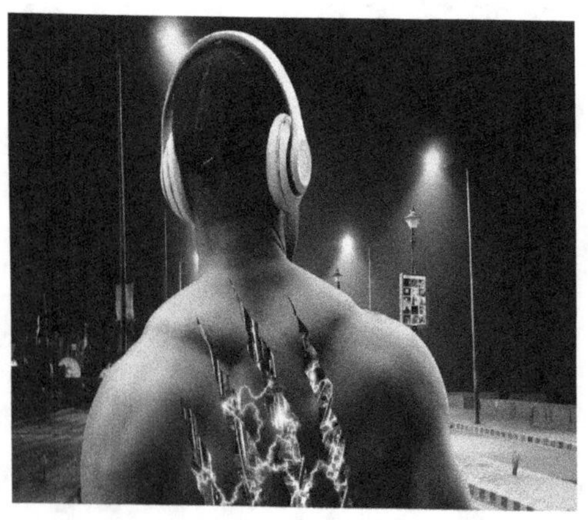

Learning how to cut body-fat the proper way is not a fun process. You have to watch what you eat, exercise more, and count your calories. The end results are always worth it. Bulking up is fun. You can eat extra calories and your clothes start to fit tighter from the newly formed muscle. Even though obesity is becoming an epidemic, there will always be some skinny people looking to bulk up.

Most superheroes are known for their super powers and bulging muscles, such as the Hulk when he picks up a truck. His muscles ripple as he exerts force.

Muscle translates to physical power and strength. People work out to feel healthier, stronger, and to live a longer life. As we have learned before, our muscle mass declines as we age. A person who carries more muscle mass will burn more calories at rest verses a person with average muscle mass. Most men and even some women who weight train want to look physically powerful.

Did you know around 3500 calories equals to one pound of body weight? Going back to the male who is 35 and has a BMR of 1706 kcal per day. The BMR and can be used as a base for muscle gain and fat loss. Once a person has established their BMR, it is crucial they stay in the positive energy balance to gain weight.

Next is to look at the person's physical activity output. Weight training sessions can burn up 200-300 calories per session depending on the intensity level. So 2-3 weight training sessions a week would be an extra 600-900 extra calories on top of 1706. That would bring the caloric intake up between 2305 and 2606 calories. I would then add an extra 400 calories to be in the positive energy balance making total caloric intake between 2705 and 3006. In order to gain muscle naturally a person must gain some body fat also.

Some experts say 1 pound of muscle for every 2-3 lbs of fat but everyone is different so there is no exact number. It is impossible to gain pure muscle mass unless the person is chemically enhanced. Chemically enhanced means the use steroids, growth hormone, clenburatol, and a list of other various drugs.

In order to lose body fat a person must follow a diet of clean eating and caloric reduction. One example of a clean protein source would be a grilled chicken breast with lemon, salt, and garlic. A bad choice would be deep-fried chicken or deep-fried, battered fish. In order to gain muscle a person must follow a higher caloric diet, so eating a cheat meal more frequently is not a bad idea. When losing body fat, it is crucial to eat clean 80-90 percent of the time but when gaining muscle a person can cheat more frequently since their calories are not as restrictive.

One of the most talked about issues when trying to add muscle mass is the protein intake and what the proper amount is. As I said before someone who is active should consume between 1.6 to 2.2 grams per kilo/day. So a person who weighs 75 kg would consume between 120-165 grams per day. If a person were to eat 3 small meals and 3 snacks a day, this would work out roughly to 20-27.5 grams of protein per meal. Using these numbers as a guide, I would round it up to 30 grams per meal.

When building muscle, it is important to also eat enough carbohydrates and fats. If a good ratio to follow is 30% protein, 50% carbohydrates, and 20% fat. If you find you're gaining too much fat, you can cut back on the carbs by 10% and increase the ratio of protein by 10%. A person eating 3000 calories a day at 30/50/20 would have the following ratio breakdowns. Protein breakdown would be 900

(3000x.30) calories and would be 225 (900/4) grams per day. The person would consume 37.5 grams per meal if they were to eat 6 times in a day. Carbohydrates would be 1500 (3000x.5) calories and would be 375 (1500/4) grams per day. The person would eat 62.5 (375/4) grams per meal if they were to eat 6 times in a day. Fats would be 600 (3000x.2) calories and would be 67 (600/9) grams per day. The person would consume 11 (67/9) grams per meal if they were to eat 6 times in a day.

After a person weight trains, it is best they consume a post-workout meal or a post-workout shake. I always have a protein and carbohydrate shake after I weight train. The shake consists of 60-80 grams of carbohydrates and 40-50 grams of protein. I never eat fat after I train as this blunts the response of insulin. Insulin is needed to shuttle the carbohydrates and protein back into the muscle.

When a person weight trains they rip muscle tissue and use up their stored glycogen inside of the muscle. So the carbohydrates are used to replenish the lost glycogen and the protein is used to repair the muscle. It is best to have a shake or meal within 30-40 minutes after training.

The last thing a person wants is to let the body starve and turn on itself for the missing nutrients. A post-workout shake for males should consist of 50-60 grams of carbs after and 40-50 grams of protein after.

A post-workout shake for females should consist of 30-40 grams of carbs and 20-30 grams of protein after. To keep things simple, any protein powder works and any fast-acting carbohydrates that is high on the GI charts.

Carbohydrates like white rice, instant oatmeal, corn-flakes, and sugars. If a person where to choose a protein food source, they should stick to faster digesting proteins like chicken, turkey, and fish.

These are just guidelines to follow but the main point to is keep a positive energy intake when trying to build muscle mass. If you are unsure of what

to eat go back and read the protein, fat, and carbohydrate chapters over again.

If you are starting to look like a good year blimp from all
the extra calories add some cardiovascular workouts
to your schedule or change the protein and carbohydrate ratio. There is no real secret to gaining
muscle but being consistent with your eating, sleep-
ing, and training.

TRAINING TIPS WHEN BULKING

Eat. Sleep. Train. Grow. That is all you should be doing when you are bulking. Opps, I forgot to mention working, arguing with your spouse, and feeding the gold fish. That is enough about everyday life activities. Here are some tips for you to follow.

1. Focus on body-part split workouts or compound movements. Compound movements are any exercise that engages two or more different joints to fully stimulate entire muscle groups and multiple muscles. Exercises such as the bench press, squat, deadlift, and chin-up.

2. Rest longer between sets and reps. When training for size, you need to train heavy and tax the muscle group. In order to do that, you must rest longer between sets and reps. Rest 60-90 seconds between sets and reps.

3. Cut back on your cardiovascular workouts but don't stop them completely. Do lower intensity cardio instead. Save all your energy for resistance training.

4. Make sure you get adequate sleep and rest days. In order to grow you must rest. Resistance training tears apart muscle tissue. Real muscle growth happens when rest.

SAMPLE DIET PLANS

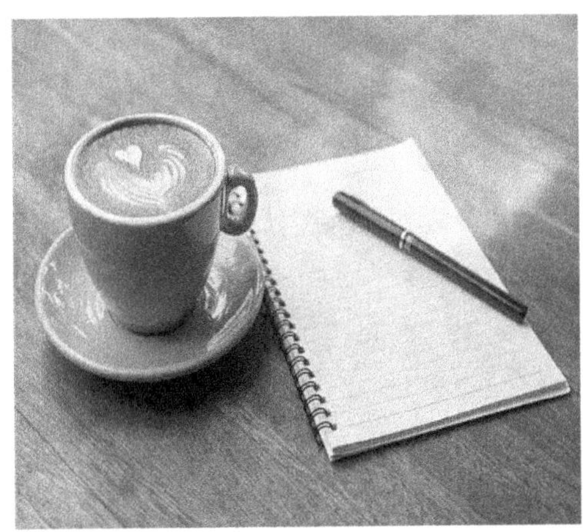

Trying to lose weight or gain muscle without the proper nutrition is like trying to drive a car with no gas. It just doesn't work. The training and the diet go hand in hand. Why not maximize your results with the proper knowledge. Here are some diet examples to get cut and to gain muscle. Do not follow them exactly, just incorporate them into your current eating plan.

TWO EXAMPLE OF DIFFERENT EATING PLANS FOR FAT LOSS

EATING PLAN 1

This is an example of a fat loss diet for a male who is moderately active, can follow a low-carbohydrate diet, and would not have as much time to eat. He would eat 3 meals and 2 snacks a day.

A cheat meal with carbs would be allowed every 4th or 5th day. This is just an example diet as you can modify it to suit your needs.

If you have a hard time following a low-carb diet, then add 1 cup of carbs to the lunch and supper. If you don't have much time for breakfast you can have snack 1 at 8:00 am and meal 1 at 3:00 pm. Please see next page.

Meal 1 8:00am	4 eggs(2 whole eggs+2 whites) 1 slice cheddar cheese 1 cup strawberries
Meal 2 12:00pm	7-8 oz of pork loin 2 cups vegetables with salad dressing
Snack 1 3:00pm	1 scoop whey protein powder 1 cup natural yogurt 1 cup bananas
Meal 6 6:00pm	7-8 oz of lean ground beef with barbecue sauce 2 cups vegetables with ranch dressing
Snack 2 8:30pm	4-5 oz chicken with jerk sauce 1 cup steamed veggies

EATING PLAN 2

This is an example a fat loss diet for a female who is moderately active and can follow a low-carb diet.

The portion sizes are smaller as females usually do not eat as much. She would eat 3 meals a day with 2 snacks and have a cheat meal with carbs every 4th or 5th day.

If you have a hard time giving up carbs then add 1/2 cup to your lunch. If you don't eat much for breakfast, you can have Snack 1 at 8:00 a.m., then have m eal 1 as snack 2 at 3:00 p.m. Please see next page.

Meal 1 8:00am	1 whole egg 1 slice cheddar cheese 1 medium sized apple
Meal 2 12:00pm	3-4 oz of chicken breast with sauce 1-1.5 cups vegetables with salad dressing
Snack 1 3:00pm	1/2 scoop whey protein powder 1 cup natural yogurt 1 cup strawberries
Meal 6 6:00pm	3-4 oz of salmon with teriyaki sauce 1-1.5 cups vegetables with ranch dressing
Snack 2 8:30pm	3-4 slices of mozzarella cheese or 1/4 cup of unsalted nuts

TWO EXAMPLE OF DIFFERENT EATING PLANS FOR GAINING MUSCLE

EATING PLAN 1

This is an example of a diet for a male who does not have as much time to eat, slower metabolism, but still wants to gain muscle mass.

He would want still to eat semi-clean as eating all fast food would result in excessive fat gain. If he did not have time to eat 2 snacks, he could incorporate weight gain shakes instead.

He would eat 3 meals and 2 snacks a day. Two cheat meals a week would be allowed. Please see next page.

Meal 1 8:00am	2 whole eggs with ketchup 2 slice whole grain toast and 2 tbs of natural peanut butter 1 medium sized pear
Meal 2 12:00pm	7-8 oz of salmon with sauce 2 cups of Caesar salad 1 medium sized potato with butter
Snack 1 3:00pm	2-3 scoop weight gain powder 2 cups milk or water 1/2 cup strawberries
Meal 3 6:00pm	7-8 oz of steak with sauce 2 cups of pasta with tomato sauce 2 cups of vegetables with salad dressing
Snack 2 8:30pm	2 cups cottage cheese or 2-3 scoops weight gain powder with 2 cups water

EATING PLAN 2

This is a variation for a female who would want to gain some muscle or who has a fast metabolism and needs to put on some body weight.

Most females want to lose weight but there are some who have an extremely fast metabolism and gaining muscle is quite a challenge.

She would have 3 meals and 2 snacks a day. Two meals would be allowed a week. Please see next page.

Meal 1 **8:00am**	2 eggs(1 whole and 1 white) 1 slice whole grain toast and 1 tbs of natural peanut butter or jam 1/2 cup grapes
Meal 2 **12:00pm**	3-4 oz turkey with sauce 1 cup of steamed broccoli 1 cup brown rice with soya sauce
Snack 1 **3:00pm**	1 scoop weigh or isolate powder 1 cup water 1 cup fruit yogurt
Meal 3 **6:00pm**	3-4 oz ground chicken with sauce 1/2 yam or small potato with cheese 1 cups of vegetables with salad dressing
Snack 2 **8:30pm**	1 protein bar or 1/4 cup nuts with 1/2 cup yogurt

RECOMMENDED FOODS

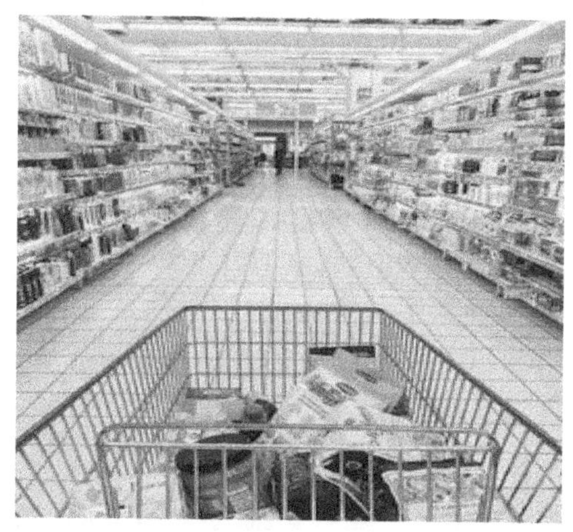

When you go grocery shopping do you often buy the wrong foods? I once went grocery shopping on empty stomach so everything looked good in the store. The chips, ice cream, frozen pizza, and the list goes on. These foods normally do not appeal to me but since I was hungry, it all looked delicious. If I did not have strong will power, I would of bought all the wrong foods.

Here is a list of foods to choose from. Remember my story and do not go shopping when you are starving.

PROTEINS

Scrambled Eggs, Whole Eggs, Chicken, Turkey, Pork,
Beef, Tofu, Tempeh, Veggie Burger, Salmon, Tuna, White
Fish, Crab, Clams, Mussels, Oysters, Shrimp, Milk,
Greek Yoghurt, Cottage Cheese, Soy Milk, Almond Milk,
Pinto Beans, Black Beans, Garbanzo Beans, Kidney
Beans, Refried Beans, Lentils, Edamame, Split Peas,
Hummus

WHOLE GRAINS & CARBS

Potatoes, Yams, Brown Rice, Wild Rice, Basmati Rice,
Oatmeal, Quinoa, Couscous, Millet, Whole Wheat
Pasta, Bran Cereal, Brown Bread, Tortillas, Barley, Farro,
Bulgur Wheat, Wheat Berries, Buck Wheat, Wheat
Berries, Buck Wheat, Corn Tortilla, Polenta, Hominy

VEGGIES

Salad Greens, Kale, Cabbage, Arugula, Parsley, Cilantro,
Basil, Broccoli, Cauliflower, Butternut Squash, Zucchini,

Acorn Squash, Pumpkin, Carrots, Beets, Turnips,
Rutabagas, Celery, Rhubarb, Radishes, Corn,
Mushrooms, Onions, Chives, Garlic, Bell Peppers,
Jalapenos, Artichokes, Brussels Sprouts, Asparagus,
Green Beans, Eggplant, Cucumber

FRUITS

Apricots, Plums, Peaches, Nectarines, Cantaloupe,
Watermelon, Honey Dew, Oranges, Melon, Tangerines,
Lemons, Limes, Papaya, Mango, Banana, Persimmons,
Kiwi, Pineapple, Apples, Pears, Grapes, Blueberries,
Blackberries, Raspberries, Cranberries, Strawberries,
Cherries, Dates, Figs, Tomatoes

HEALTHY FATS

Sour Cream, Butter, Cream Cheese, Cheese, Salad
Dressing, Avocado, Olive Oil, Coconut Oil, Seeds, Nuts,
Nut Butter, Flax Seed, Mayonnaise, Dark Chocolate,
Cocoa Powder

WHAT IS FLEXIBLE DIETING

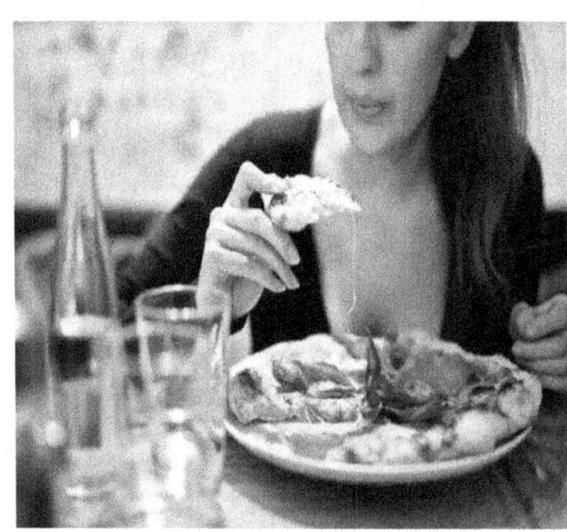

Flexible dieting is not an actual diet. It's more of a lifestyle. It promotes the notion that there are no "bad foods" and allows you to choose any food, as long as it fits within your macronutrient needs. Sounds good? Read on.

It puts the control in the hands of the dieter, meaning there are no meal plans or food restrictions that need to be followed. You may ask yourself, how do you lose weigh then?

To use flexible dieting in your lifestyle, you can start by using 2 different measures. I use TDEE and BMR as you have read earlier. TDEE is the total calories burned daily and BMR is calories you burn at rest. If a person is eating well over there TDEE and starting to exercise, I get them to follow their TDEE as a start. In flexible dieting you can eat whatever you want but as long as you stay within your caloric intake(TDEE). The person will lose some weight but they will eventually hit a plateau. When this happens, I get them to follow their BMR. This is much lower than their TDEE and will create more fat loss. The reason being is that there is a greater calorie deficit when using the BMR verses the TDEE. The person also starts to build more muscle mass through resistance training and this burns more calories at rest. Your body becomes like furnace for burning calories.

I also like to give some fat loss recommendations to people in order them to lose fat faster. In flexible dieting, you eat the foods you enjoy and still lose weight with the proper combination of cardio and resistance training. The weight loss is slower but the person gets to follow a diet that is less restrictive.

The Weight Watchers app is an example of flexible dieting. The user can eat foods they like but they have to follow a point system. Higher caloric foods are more points verses vegetables which are lower in points. Weight watchers is the number one weight loss system. I wonder why? Flexible dieting. It works.

WHAT DO YOU DO WHEN YOU HIT A PLATEAU?

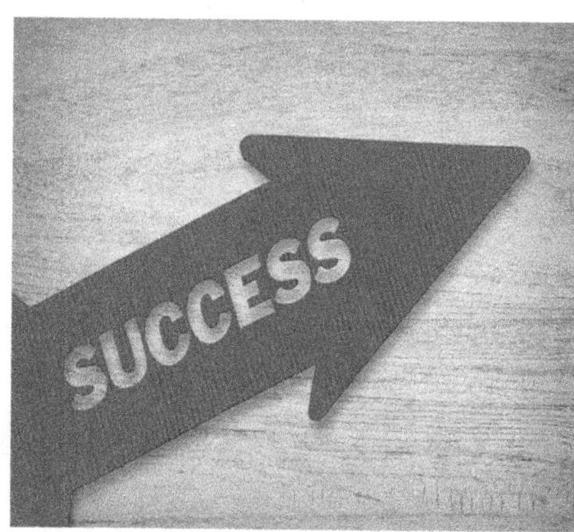

No one likes to hit a plateau. A plateau is defined as a state of little or no change following a period of activity or progress. There are 2 different scenarios I am going to mention here. One is when a person bulks up and the other is when a person is cutting bodyfat. Let's go over scenario one.

The bulk up process is going well as planned. You are lifting heavier weights, getting proper rest, and eating well over your TDEE. Your girlfriend and family are starting to complain about the gas you are expelling from eating copious amounts of protein. After 10 weeks of bulking up, you have successfully gained 15 lbs of muscle and fat. You plan for another 10 lbs and then nothing happens in the next 2-3 weeks. What should you do next?

What is happening in this scenario is common. Your body has natural genetic limitations for gaining muscle and size. If you were to do anabolic steroids you could easily gain another 10 lbs in addition to the 15 lbs. Always try to stay natural as this is the safest route. Even with supplements like creatine, AKG, and test boosters, you will still hit a plateau. I will go over supplements in the next chapter.

In order to get over this plateau, I would start to cut body fat for 2 weeks or implement a cutting phase for 8-10 weeks. This shocks the body with the change in caloric intake and training. I prefer not to go into detail on how the metabolism works as you might fall asleep. After the cutting phase you can go back to bulking for another 8-10 weeks. This theory works as I use to bulk up for 8-10 weeks then cut for 10 weeks when I was preparing for a competition. The end result was a freaky looking human being.

Now let's move unto scenario 2. What to do if you hit a plateau during the cutting phase. The reason you hit a plateau is because your body has a natural weight it likes to stay at. To go above it or below it, the body will stall and fight back to keep it at a comfort zone. I like to attack weight loss in increments of 10 lbs. This depends on how much body fat a person has to lose. Here are some tricks I use to fight a plateau.

1. Increase Or Change Up The Cardio
By increasing the cardio you are burning more calories which will create a bigger calorie deficit. If a person is doing HITT for 30 minutes on a bike I get them to do 30 minutes on a treadmill keeping it at regular pace.

2. Schedule One or Two Refeed Meals
I like to do this with my clients only if they are close to hitting their body weight and have been staying at

a caloric deficit. For a reffeed day they get to eat one or 2 large carbohydrate meals in order to shock their metabolism. When you have been in a calorie deficit for a period of time, your body goes into a starvation mode and tries to hold onto it's body fat. By giving your body a surplus of calories, it will trick the brain into going back into a fat burning mode.

3. In the quest to lose body fat, muscle mass is also lost. To combat this a person could do one or 2 weeks of bulking and then resume their fat loss attack. The same theory works with cutting also. When you hit a plateau, change the training and go into a caloric surplus to shock the body.

SUPPLEMENT RECOMMENDATIONS

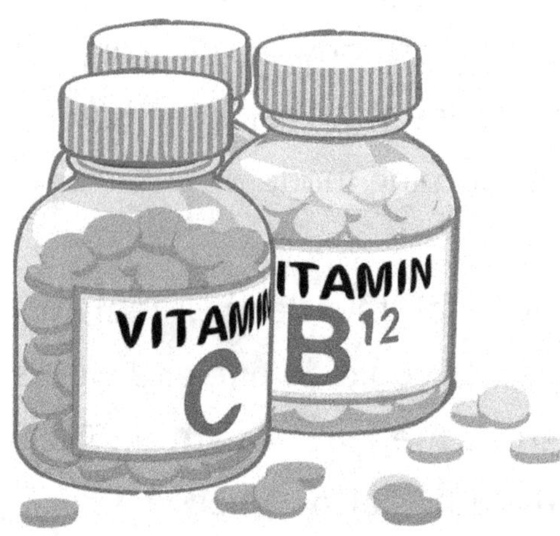

Whey protein. Branched chained amino acids. Vitamins. Weight gainer shakes. The list goes on and on. The supplement industry is a billion dollar business and keeps growing every year.

I use to own a supplement business and I have taken supplements over the last 20 years. My parents are health nuts so we often discuss the latest trends in this industry.

With so many different types of supplements out there, it is easy to get confused.

When it comes to vitamin recommendations, it is best to seek advice from a dietitian, certified nutritionist, or naturopath. I will be going over what supplements are best to use when cutting or bulking.

SUPPLEMENTS FOR CUTTING

1. Protein powder

One of the main uses of this supplement is to help rebuild muscle tissue. Protein powder is also a base supplement when it comes to either cutting, maintaining, or bulking. Instead of eating 6-7 chicken breasts a day to get your protein requirements, people often use this supplement instead. It is very versatile and you can mix it in a shake or have it with some yogurt for a tasty snack.

There are different types of protein powder. Here are the 3 most common types. One is not particularly better than the other but it depends on personal preference. I use whey concentration when I am cutting since it keeps me full longer. The isolate and hydrolyze go through my system faster. I use isolate when I am bulking since I am full most of the time.

Whey Concentrate

This form of powder typically has a low level of fat and cholesterol content when compared to regular whey protein. It's also higher in carbohydrates which come in the form of lactose – a sugar compound derived from glucose, most commonly found in milk. Whey concentrate is also seen as the cheapest and most common form of protein powder on the market today.

The protein levels in whey concentrate can also vary greatly with companies offering powders or supplements containing anywhere between 40-90% protein content per serving, depending on the source. Concentrate will also have a higher level of lactose within the compound, which will result in an increase in both sugar and carbohydrate levels in the protein. People who are lactose intolerant should stay away from this type of protein.

Whey Isolate

This is usually processed and refined in a process that will remove the fat and the lactose from the powder, making isolate one of the leanest protein powders by trade and comprising of over 90% protein content per serving. Whey isolate is more expensive than regular whey and concentrate.

Some isolate powders are lactose free which makes it a suitable product for many people who have an allergy to dairy or are vegan or vegetarian.

Hydrolyzed Whey

This is a whey protein that has gone through the process of hydrolysis. Hydrolysis is comprised of two terms: Hydro- meaning water, and – lysis which means to remove. Whey protein that undergoes the hydrolysis process simply is whey protein that has had the addition of water into the substance to allow for the protein to be broken down. The sole purpose is to be metabolized and absorbed much easier.

This protein is superior to whey but is more expensive. It's also important to know that hydrolyzed whey is also typically less allergenic when compared to other forms of whey protein.

2. Fat Burners
Fat burners can help support fat loss by enhancing metabolism, maintaining healthy appetite, and minimizing cravings. They can also optimize workout potential by increasing energy and focus. A person must be following a proper diet and training in order to see results.

Fat burner are good to use if you have that last 10 lbs of fat to lose or you need a kick start to get going. I would not suggest using fat burners if you have over 100 lbs to lose.

Fat burners are generally safe but if not recommended for people who have high blood pressure and heart conditions.

The best fat burner on the market is the ECA stack. This is a combination of ephedrine, caffeine, and aspirin. All 3 of these supplements work synergistically together. I won't go into dosages here as you can find that information on the internet. Just be smart about the dosages as taking excessive amounts can cause some serious health problems.

I have used all types of fat burners and found the ECA stack to be the most effective for burning fat. Some fat burners are a waste of money as they do nothing.

3. Pre-workouts
Pre-workout supplements are designed to support increased energy, focus, and endurance in the gym.

Most of these supplements contain caffeine, creatine, and different types of amino acids. The are few that contain no caffeine or stimulants. People often take them before weight training in order to squeeze out those extra few repetitions.

If you are already taking a fat burner with caffeine, it is safer to use a non-stimulant pre-workout. Excessive amounts of caffeine can cause high blood pressure and adrenal gland burn out.

4. Creatine
Creatine is the number one supplement for improving performance in the gym. This supplement is used in order to gain muscle, enhance strength and improve exercise performance.

I won't go into the exact science on how it works but creatine helps to replenish your ATP stores. ATP is the currency your body uses for energy. By doing this you can run faster and lift heavier.

There are a few different types of creatine on the market, but monohydrate is the most common form. During a cutting phase, it is best to stay away from monohydrate. What I would use is creatine hydrochloride or trimaltate. Monohydrate causes excessive bloating which will make you look like a marshmallow. The other 2 will cause less water retention giving you a tighter look.

5. L-Arginine
This supplement is supposed to enhance blood flow, energy and recovery. Enhanced blood flow equals a greater pump. L-Arginine is a nonessential amino acid that is also involved in the production of nitric oxide, a biological signal that regulates blood flow.

There has been some debate if this supplement is worth taking. This is something you have to figure out yourself. Do not use L-arginine if you are planning to use ephedrine. They cancel out each other. People with heart conditions should check with their doctors before using this product.

I have used L-arginine and have noticed increased pumps.

6. Glutamine

Glutamine is one of the most common amino acids found in your muscles. Did you know over 61% of skeletal muscle is Glutamine?

During intense training, Glutamine levels are greatly depleted in your body, which decreases strength, stamina and recovery. It could take up to 5-6 days for Glutamine levels to return to normal. Some studies have shown that L-Glutamine supplementation can minimize breakdown of muscle and improve protein metabolism.

This is another hit and miss supplement. Some people swear by it and others think it is useless.

I have used glutamine for years and have noticed less muscle soreness. Supplements can get expensive, so pick and chose what is best for you.

SUPPLEMENTS FOR BULKING

1. Protein Powder

I won't talk again about the different types of protein powder but it can be used during bulking and cutting to get that extra needed protein.

2. Weight Gainers

If you have trouble getting the calories needed to support muscle growth, then a high calorie, high protein weight gainer may be the answer you need to build rock solid, muscle mass.

Instead of eating 7 times a day, you could supplement with 3 weight gain shakes to reach your target caloric intake.

I have used weight gainer shakes during my bulking phase with great results. If I were to eat 5000 calories a day, 2000 calories would come from shakes and the other 3000 calories would be from food.

3. Creatine

Creatine can be used for both bulking and cutting. You can use monohydrate during the bulking phase. If you prefer to be less bloated and hold less water, use the other types I mentioned before.

4. Pre-Workouts

Pre-workouts can be used during both phases. If you are planning to use creatine and L-arginine during the bulking phase, there is no need to use a pre-workout. Most pre-workouts are a combination of caffeine, l-arginine, and creatine.

5. L-Arginine

This wonder supplement can be used during bulking and cutting. Use only what is recommend. More is not going to produce faster results.

6. Glutamine

I use glutamine year round during both phases. My strength is always better during the bulking phase so I am able to lift heavier. Lifting heavier results in more torn muscles. Glutamine is a protein(amino acid) so it will aid in muscle repair.

SAMPLE WORKOUT ROUTINES

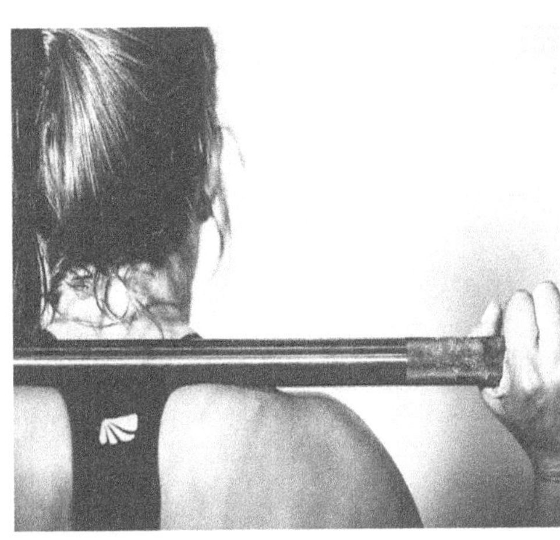

Oh yeah! We have now made it to the workouts. This is my favourite part. I love to design workout programs for people regardless of their injuries and age. When you have been a personal trainer for over 20 years, program designing becomes like a second nature to me.

Here are a few different programs that you can do at your home or in the gym. These are great starter workouts to get you going. If you are unsure of any exercises, google it.

Full body workouts are the best for burning calories and for fat loss. Body part splits are done when a person is trying to gain more muscle. Bodybuilders train this way to gain muscle mass. I have included both types of programs so you can see how to structure your workouts and exercises.

 Always consult a physician or doctor before starting any type of exercise program.

Full Body Workout – Home

Men

1. Warm up for 5-6 minutes

2. One arm dumbbell rows – 1x12, 1x10, 1x8 reps

3. Dumbbell plie squats – 1x12, 1x10, 1x8 reps

4. Dumbbell bench press flat – 1x12, 1x10, 1x8 reps

5. Running on spot for 1 minute

6. Dumbbell stiff legged dead lifts – 1x12, 1x10, 1x8 reps

7. Dumbbell calf rocks – 1x20, 1x20, 1x20 reps

8. Dumbbell shoulder press – 1x12, 1x10, 1x8 reps

9. Bench dips – 1x12, 1x10, 1x8 reps

10. One arm dumbbell concentration curls – 1x12, 1x10, 1x8 reps

11. Cool down for 5-6 minutes

12. Static stretching

Full Body Workout – Home

Women

1. Warm up for 5-6 minutes

2. Dumbbell plie squats – 1x15, 1x12, 1x10 reps

3. Dumbbell one arm rows -1x15, 1x12, 1x10 reps

4. Jumping jacks – 1x20, 1x20, 1x20 reps

5. Dumbbell flat bench presses - 1x15, 1x12, 1x10 reps

6. Dumbbell stiff legged dead lifts - 1x15, 1x12, 1x10 reps

7. Jumping jacks - 1x20, 1x20, 1x20 reps

8. Dumbbell calf rocks - 1x15, 1x12, 1x10 reps

9. Dumbbell upright rows - 1x15, 1x12, 1x10 reps

10. Dumbbell triceps kickbacks - 1x15, 1x12, 1x10 reps for each side

11. Dumbbell biceps curls - 1x15, 1x12, 1x10 reps

12. Cool down - 5-6 minutes

13. Static stretching after

Full Body Workouts – Gym

Men And Women

Week 1

Sunday: Rest or walking for 20 minutes

Monday: Workout 1 (full body workout)

Tuesday: Rest

Wednesday: Cardio + core (abs)

Thursday: Workout 2 (full body workout)

Friday: Rest

Saturday: Cardio + core (abs)

Monday

Workout 1

1. Warm up for 5-6 minutes on a cardio machine

2. Lat pull down to front – 1x12, 1x10, 1x8 reps

3. Machine leg press – 1x12, 1x10, 1x8 reps

4. Machine back row – 1x12, 1x10, 1x8 reps

5. Machine bench press – 1x12, 1x10, 1x8 reps

6. Lying prone machine hamstring curls – 1x12, 1x10, 1x8 reps

7. Machine shoulder press – 1x12, 1x10, 1x8 reps

8. Seated adductor machine – 1x15, 1x12, 1x10 reps

9. Cool down for 5-6 minutes on a cardio machine

10. Static stretching or use my stretching app

www.pursefitness.com

Wednesday

Cardio – 25 minutes

1. Bike – 12.5 minutes

2. Treadmill – 12.5 minutes

Core

1. Bird dogs - 1 x12, 1x12 reps

2. Seated leg lifts – 1x15, 1x15 for each side

3. Cable crunches - 1x15, 1x15 reps

4. Standing medicine ball twists – 1 minute

Thursday

Workout 2

1. Warm up for 5-6 minutes on a cardio machine

2. Reverse grip bar pull downs – 1x15, 1x12, 1x10 reps

3. Seated machine leg extensions – 1x15, 1x12, 1x10 reps

4. Pulley low grip back rows – 1x15, 1x12, 1x10 reps

5. Flat dumbbell chest fly – 1x15, 1x12, 1x10 reps

6. Seated upright hamstring curls – 1x15, 1x12, 1x10 reps

7. Dumbbell side laterals – 1x15, 1x12, 1x10 reps

8. Seal jacks – 1x15, 1x15 reps

9. Machine triceps extension – 1x15, 1x12, 1x10 reps

10. Machine biceps curls – 1x15, 1x10 reps

11. Cool down for 5-6 minutes on a cardio machine

12. Static stretching or use my stretching app

www.pursefitness.com

Saturday

Cardio – 25 minutes

1. Elliptical – 12.5 minutes

2. Rowing – 12.5 minutes

Core

1. Hold superman – 1x15, 1x15 seconds

2. Standing bicycle crunches – 1x15, 1x15 reps

3. Oblique cable twists – 1x15, 1x15 each side

Body- Part Split Workouts – Gym

Men

Sunday: Cardio + core

Monday: Back + hamstrings

Tuesday: Chest + triceps

Wednesday: Rest day

Thursday: Shoulders + biceps + forearms + core

Friday: Quadriceps + calves + traps

Saturday: Rest day

Sunday

Cardio

1. Bike or tread mile - 25 minutes

Core

1. Bird dog - 1 x12, 1x12 reps for each side

2. Flutter kicks - 1 x 15, 1x15, 1x15 reps

3. Dumbbell push crunches - 1x 15, 1x15, 1x15 reps

4. Bent knee side planks - 1 x 20-30 seconds each side

Monday

Back

1. Assisted pull-ups or pull-ups - 1x10, 1x8, 1x6 reps

2. Reverse grip lat pull downs - 1x10, 1x8, 1x6 reps

3. Bent over barbell rows- 1x10, 1x8, 1x6 reps

4. Close grip low pulley row - 1x10, 1x8, 1x6 reps

Hamstrings

1. Lying hamstring curl machine - 1x10, 1x8, 1x6 reps

2. Barbell Romanian dead lifts - 1x10, 1x8, 1x6 reps

Tuesday

Chest

1. Incline barbell bench press - 1x10, 1x8, 1x6 reps

2. Barbell bench press - 1x10, 1x8, 1x6 reps

3. Dumbbell pullover - 1x10, 1x8, 1x6 reps

Triceps

1. Bar pulley push downs - 1x10, 1x8, 1x6 reps

2. Cable rope overhead triceps extension - 1x10, 1x8 reps

3. Lying barbell triceps extension - 1x10, 1x8 reps

Thursday

Shoulders

1. Barbell seated shoulder press - 1x10, 1x8, 1x6 reps

2. Dumbbell lateral raise - 1x10, 1x8, 1x6 reps

3. Dumbbell rear delt row - 1x10, 1x8, 1x6 reps

Biceps

1. Barbell biceps curl - 1x10, 1x8, 1x6 reps

2. Machine preacher curls - 1x10, 1x8, 1x6 reps

Forearms

1. Behind the body wrist curls - 1x10, 1x8 reps

2. Reverse grip barbell bicep curls - 1x10, 1x8 reps

Core

1. Same core as Sunday workout

Friday

Quadriceps

1. Leg press - 1x10, 1x8, 1x6, 1x4 reps

2. Barbell full squats - 1x10, 1x8, 1x6, 1x4 reps

3. Leg extension machine - 1x10, 1x8, 1x6, 1x4 reps

Calves

1. Seated calf raises machine- 1x12, 1x10, 1x8 reps

2. Standing calf raises - 1x12, 1x10, 1x8 reps

Traps

1. Dumbbell shrugs - 1x10, 1x8, 1x6 reps

Body- Part Split Workouts – Gym

Women

Sunday: Cardio + core

Monday: Back + hamstrings

Tuesday: Chest + triceps

Wednesday: Rest day

Thursday: Shoulders + biceps + cardio

Friday: Quadriceps + calves +core

Saturday: Rest day

Sunday

Cardio

1. Bike or tread mile - 30 minutes

Core

1. Bird dog - 1 x12, 1x12 reps for each side

2. Flutter kicks - 1 x 15, 1x15, 1x15 reps

3. Dumbbell push crunches - 1x 15, 1x15, 1x15 reps

4. Bent knee side planks - 1 x 20-30 seconds each side

Monday

Back

1. Assisted pull-ups or pull-ups - 1x10, 1x8, 1x6 reps

2. Reverse grip lat pull downs - 1x10, 1x8, 1x6 reps

3. Bent over barbell rows- 1x10, 1x8, 1x6 reps

4. Close grip low pulley row - 1x10, 1x8, 1x6 reps

Hamstrings

1. Lying hamstring curl machine - 1x10, 1x8, 1x6 reps

2. Barbell Romanian dead lifts - 1x10, 1x8, 1x6 reps

Tuesday

Chest

1. Barbell bench press - 1x10, 1x8, 1x6 reps

2. Incline dumbbell flys – 1x10, 1x8, 1x6 reps

3. Dumbbell pullover - 1x10, 1x8, 1x6 reps

Triceps

1. Bar pulley push downs - 1x10, 1x8, 1x6 reps

2. Cable rope overhead triceps extension - 1x10, 1x8 reps

3. Lying barbell triceps extension - 1x10, 1x8 reps

Thursday

Shoulders

1. Barbell seated shoulder press - 1x10, 1x8, 1x6 reps

2. Dumbbell lateral raise - 1x10, 1x8, 1x6 reps

3. Dumbbell rear delt row - 1x10, 1x8, 1x6 reps

Biceps

1. Barbell biceps curl - 1x10, 1x8, 1x6 reps

2. Machine preacher curls - 1x10, 1x8, 1x6 reps

Cardio

-same cardio as Sunday

Friday

Quadriceps

1. Leg press - 1x10, 1x8, 1x6, 1x4 reps

2. Barbell full squats - 1x10, 1x8, 1x6, 1x4 reps

3. Leg extension machine - 1x10, 1x8, 1x6, 1x4 reps

Calves

1. Seated calf raises machine- 1x12, 1x10, 1x8 reps

2. Standing calf raises - 1x12, 1x10, 1x8 reps

Core

- same core as Sunday workout

CONCLUSION

Now you see why it is a challenge to get started on the proper path to getting that physique you have always wanted. With so much information out there, it is easy to get confused. Even if you do utilize all the proper information from this book, you still have to stay consistent to get results.

Being consistent is one of the best ways to get the results you want. Like I mentioned before, you put in 100%, you get 100% back. If you really want to fast track your progress, hire a reputable personal trainer.

Good luck with your journey on becoming the fittest or the most muscular human being!

ABOUT THE AUTHOR

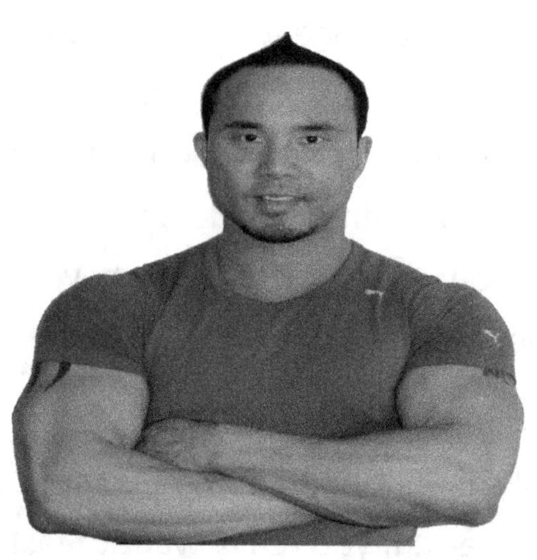

Paul Nam has been in the fitness industry and a personal trainer for over 20 years. He started bodybuilding at the age of 18 and became the Junior Mackenzie Bodybuilding champion at 19. He has since then competed in over 25 bodybuilding, fitness, and martial arts competitions. He has trained in Olympic style boxing, Brazilian jui-jitsu, muay thai, wrestling, and holds a red belt in tae kwon do.

Paul owns a fitness studio in Toronto, builds mobile training apps, and writes books. He is also focusing on bringing new fitness products to the world.